Dr. Dee Dee Dynamo's™
HyperTension Take Down!

COLORING & ACTIVITY BOOK

Written by
Oneeka Williams, M.D.

Illustrated by Valerie Bouthyette

Positive Health Series

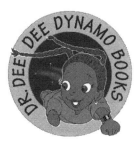

ISBN 978-0-9983045-7-1
Printed in the United States

DR. DEE DEE DYNAMO'S
5 HABITS OF POSITIVITY

1. There is ALWAYS a solution, WORK to find it!

2. CONVERT a limit into an OPPORTUNITY.

3. KEEP the POSITIVE, DISCARD the negative.

4. Find PURPOSE in CARING for others.

5. Be THANKFUL and BELIEVE!

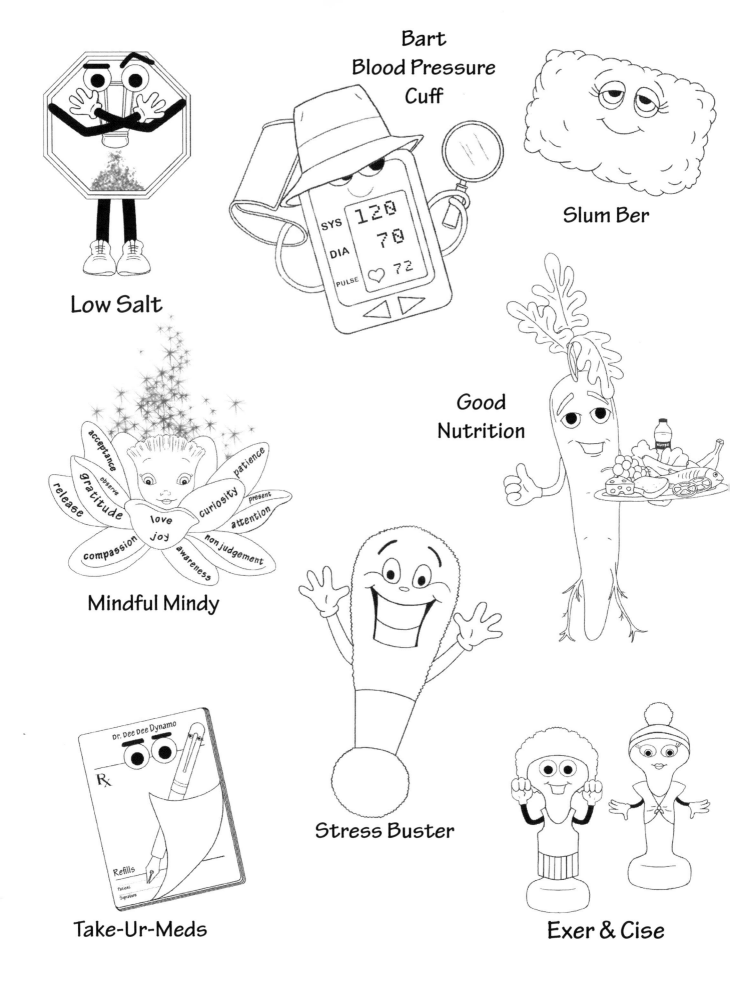

Low Salt

Bart
Blood Pressure
Cuff

Slum Ber

Mindful Mindy

Good
Nutrition

Stress Buster

Take-Ur-Meds

Exer & Cise

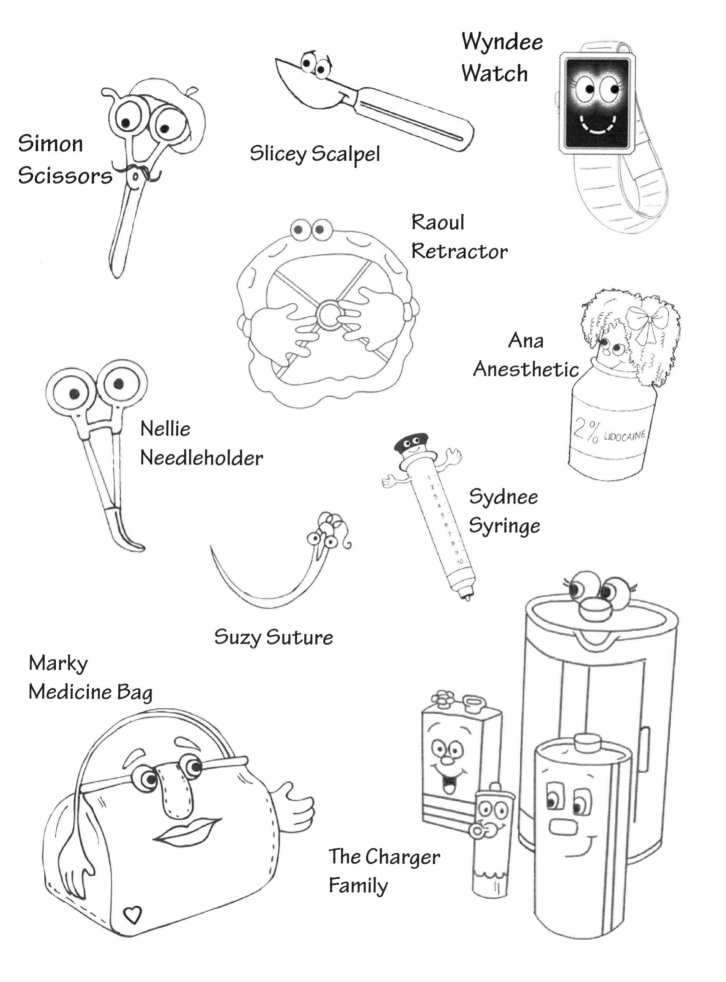

Simon Scissors

Slicey Scalpel

Wyndee Watch

Raoul Retractor

Ana Anesthetic

2% LIDOCAINE

Nellie Needleholder

Sydnee Syringe

Suzy Suture

Marky Medicine Bag

The Charger Family

Conga Line! Conga Line! Everybody do the Conga Line!!!!

Take a Positivity Pause and come join us at the annual Island of Positivity Beach Party on Feel Good Beach! The Dynamo kids are leading the festive Conga Line!

Fluffy clouds are dancing in the sky to the conga beat and the sun is beaming with joy.

It is a perfect day!

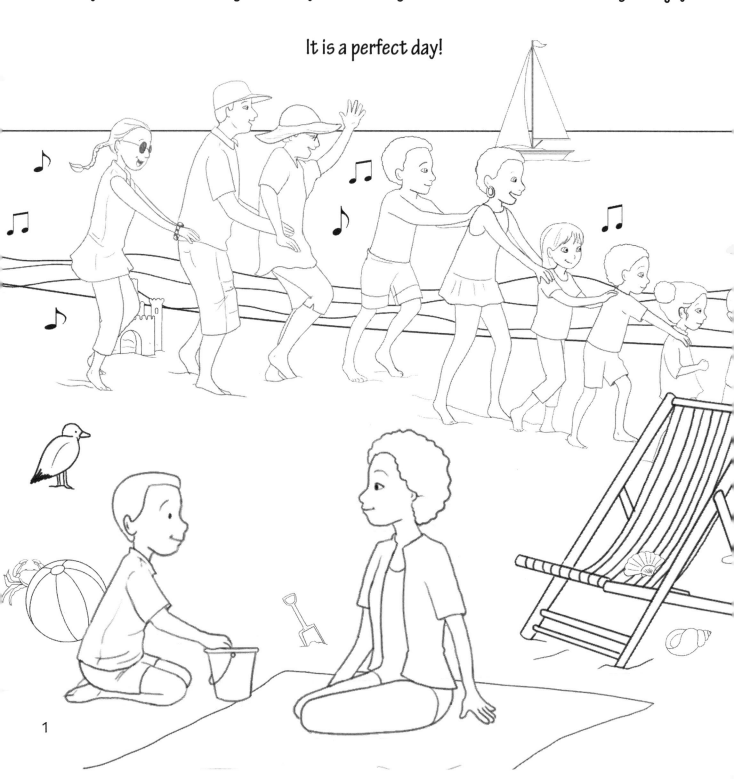

Dr. Dee Dee Dynamo is a 9-year-old girl super surgeon, born with super powers of positivity and electrical energy. She fixes any problem with her gifted hands and has a great team that goes with her on missions. Her home is on the Island of Positivity where she lives with her parents and extended family.

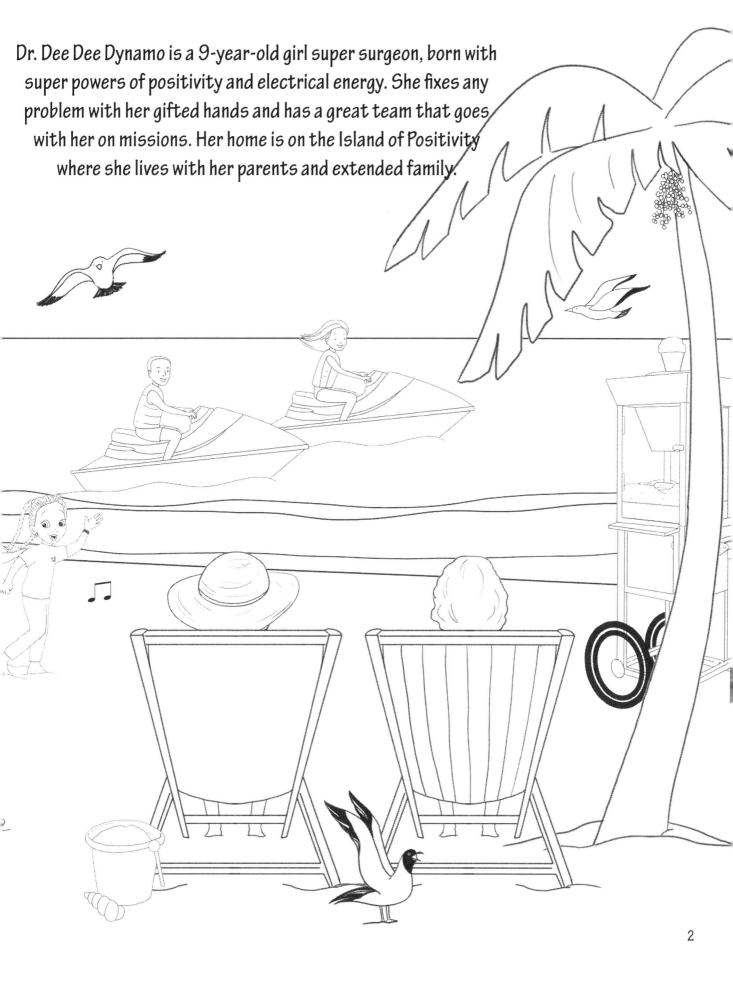

Mommy Dynamo is putting the finishing touches on the picnic table and asks, "Where are Grandma B and Granddad Willy? They should have been here by now."

Daddy Dynamo says, "Grandma B has been up all night and she was almost done cooking when I left home. I'm sure they are on their way."

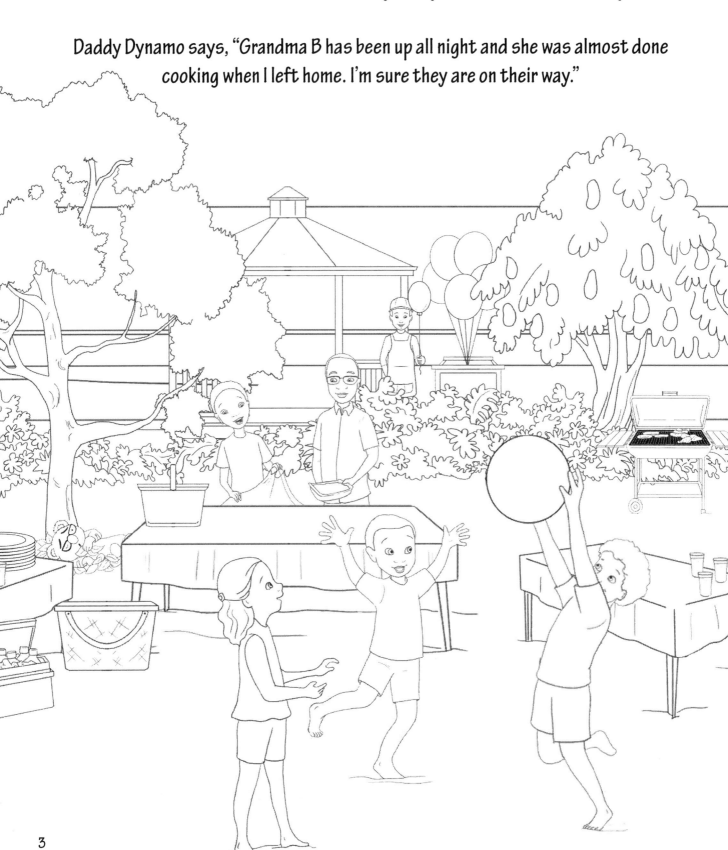

"Yum Yum!" says cousin Lukas. "I love Grandma B's macaroni and cheese. Her barbecue chicken and potato salad are so delicious. My mouth is watering!"

Kyle, Dr. Dee Dee Dynamo's very grumpy assistant, complains. "All this fuss and noise are so annoying. I just want to sleep."

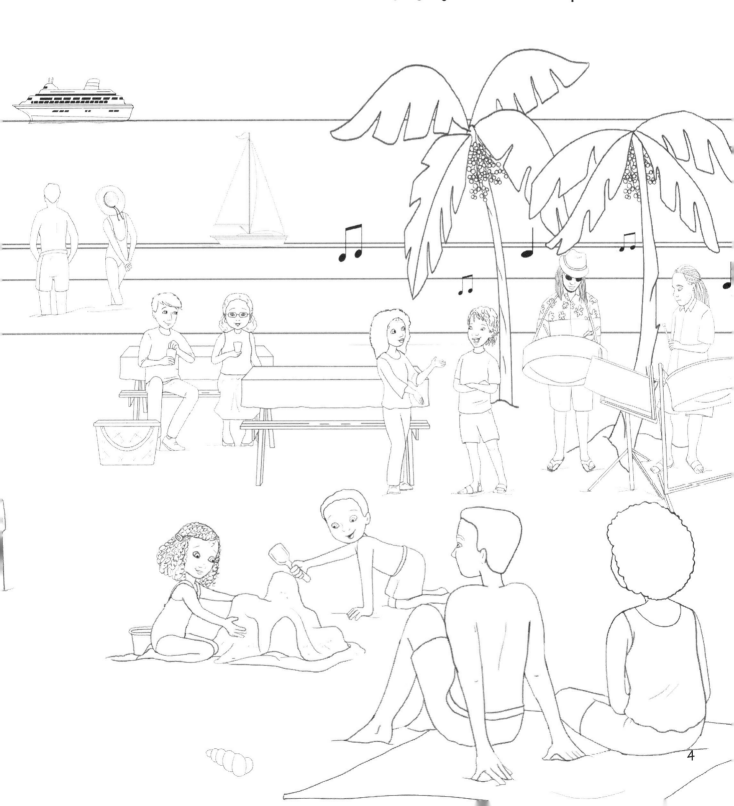

4

WAHOO! WAHOO! WAHOO!

Gordon's alarm makes everyone stop. Gordon the Gullible Globe has
super sensitive ears and can hear whenever someone in the Universe is in distress.

"What is it, Gordon?" asks Dr. Dee Dee Dynamo.

"It's Grandma B," Gordon replies. "Her insides are moaning and groaning."

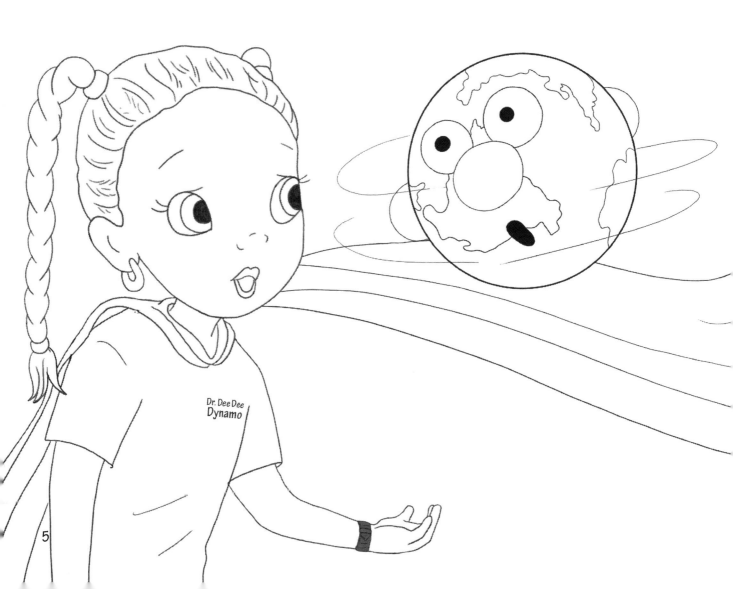

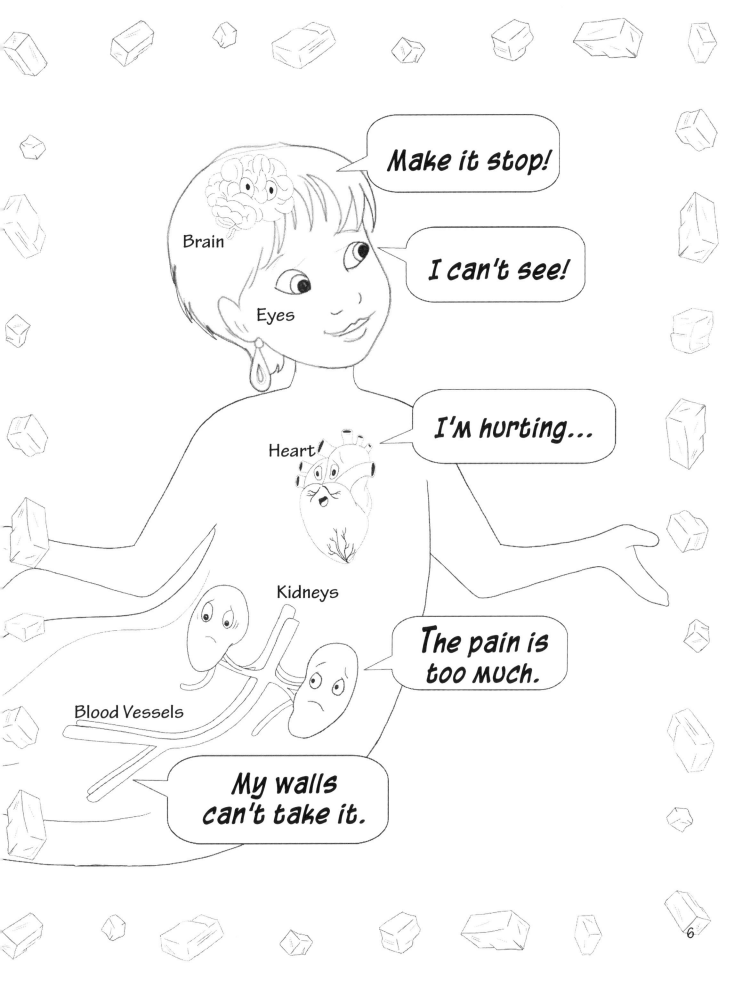

"Oh boy," says Dr. Dee Dee. "It sounds like that monster Hyper Tension is causing trouble again. We must go to Grandma B quickly."

Dr. Dee Dee looks at her watch Wyndee.
Wyndee measures Dr. Dee Dee's electrical charge.
She launches into the air and says, "I'm CHARGED UP and Ready To Go!"

"Come on Freeda!" says Dr. Dee Dee, singing happily as her fingers begin to tingle!

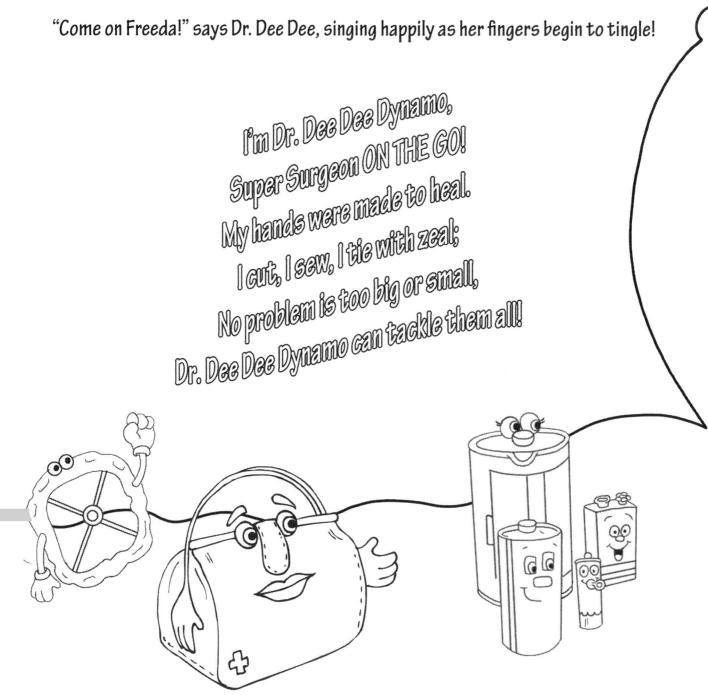

I'm Dr. Dee Dee Dynamo,
Super Surgeon ON THE GO!
My hands were made to heal.
I cut, I sew, I tie with zeal;
No problem is too big or small,
Dr. Dee Dee Dynamo can tackle them all!

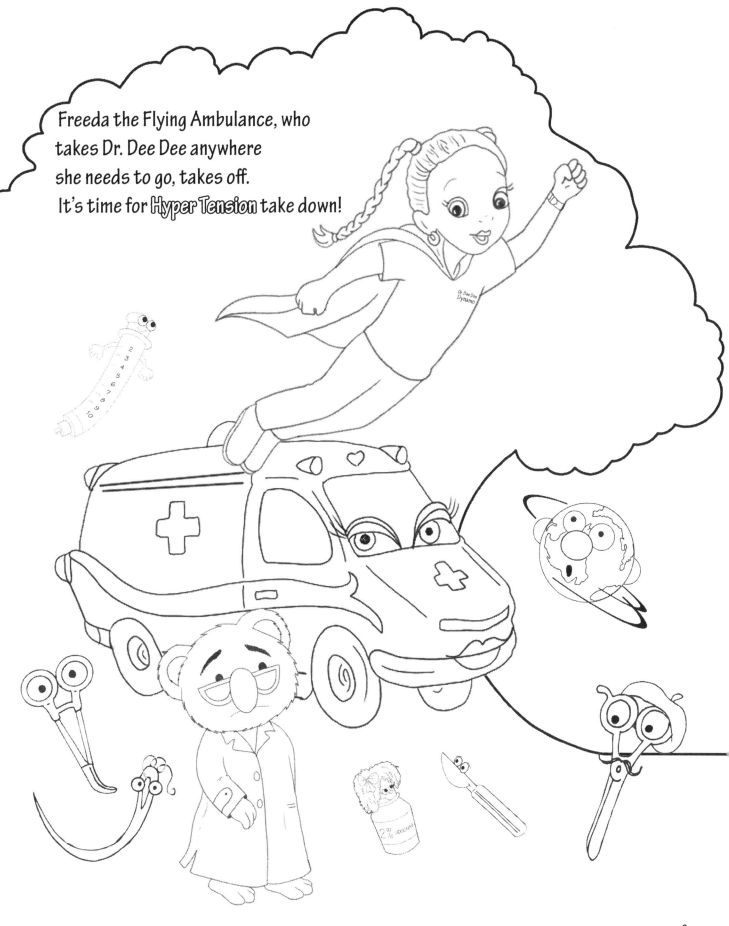

Freeda the Flying Ambulance, who
takes Dr. Dee Dee anywhere
she needs to go, takes off.
It's time for Hyper Tension take down!

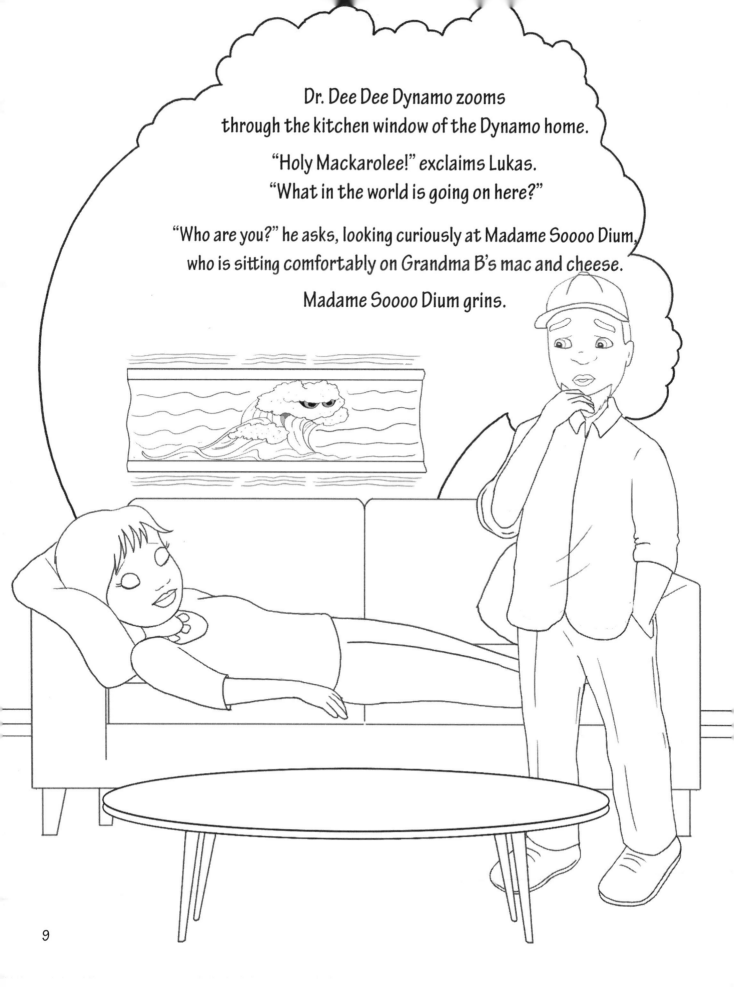

Dr. Dee Dee Dynamo zooms
through the kitchen window of the Dynamo home.

"Holy Mackarolee!" exclaims Lukas.
"What in the world is going on here?"

"Who are you?" he asks, looking curiously at Madame Soooo Dium,
who is sitting comfortably on Grandma B's mac and cheese.

Madame Soooo Dium grins.

9

I'm Madame Soooo Dium
HT's best friend
I make food taste super good
I'll hang with HT till the end.

Before the fridge
In days of old
I kept food from going bad
Cause there was no way to keep it cold.

Now you don't like me
It's so unfair
But I'm here to stay
I'm everywhere!

Watch me Bling
Watch me Nay Nay
Watch me Bling Bling,
Watch me Nay Nay!

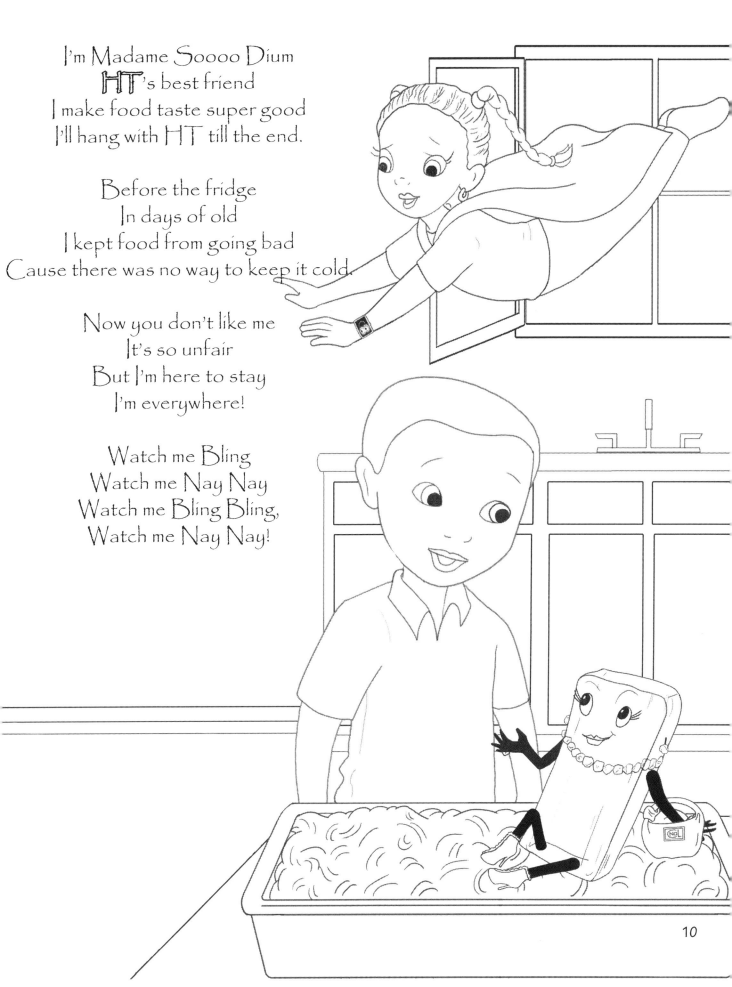

10

Dr. Dee Dee opens Marky Medicine Bag and Bart Blood Pressure Cuff pops out like a jack-in-the-box! He is always on the lookout for HT, also known as high blood pressure. He is ready for this mission! He places his cuff around Grandma B's arm.

The reading is very high.

$$\frac{180}{110}$$

SYS 180
DIA 110
PULSE ♥ 94

HT is crashing through Grandma B's body and scares Lukas. HT says,

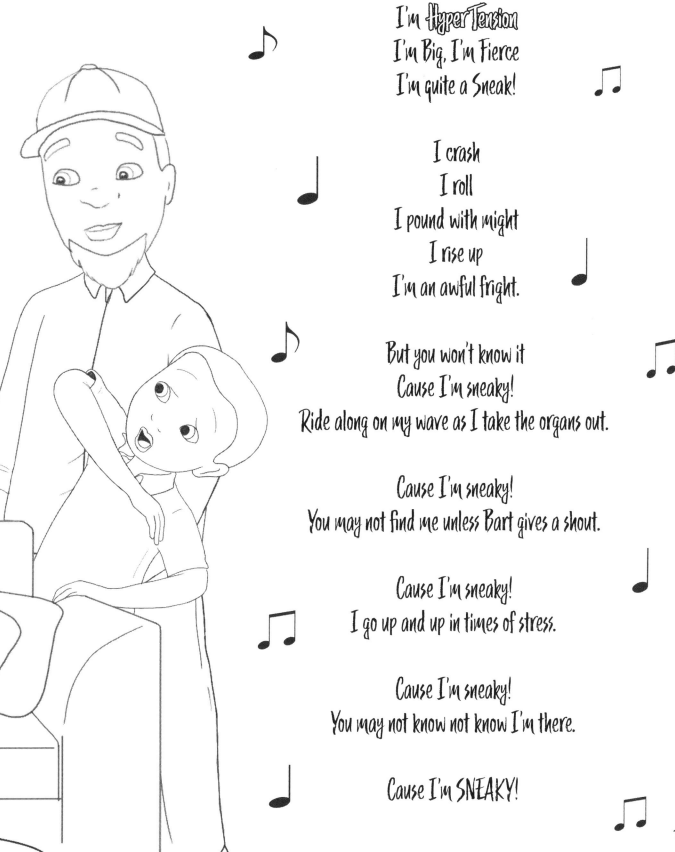

I'm *HyperTension*
I'm Big, I'm Fierce
I'm quite a Sneak!

I crash
I roll
I pound with might
I rise up
I'm an awful fright.

But you won't know it
Cause I'm sneaky!
Ride along on my wave as I take the organs out.

Cause I'm sneaky!
You may not find me unless Bart gives a shout.

Cause I'm sneaky!
I go up and up in times of stress.

Cause I'm sneaky!
You may not know not know I'm there.

Cause I'm SNEAKY!

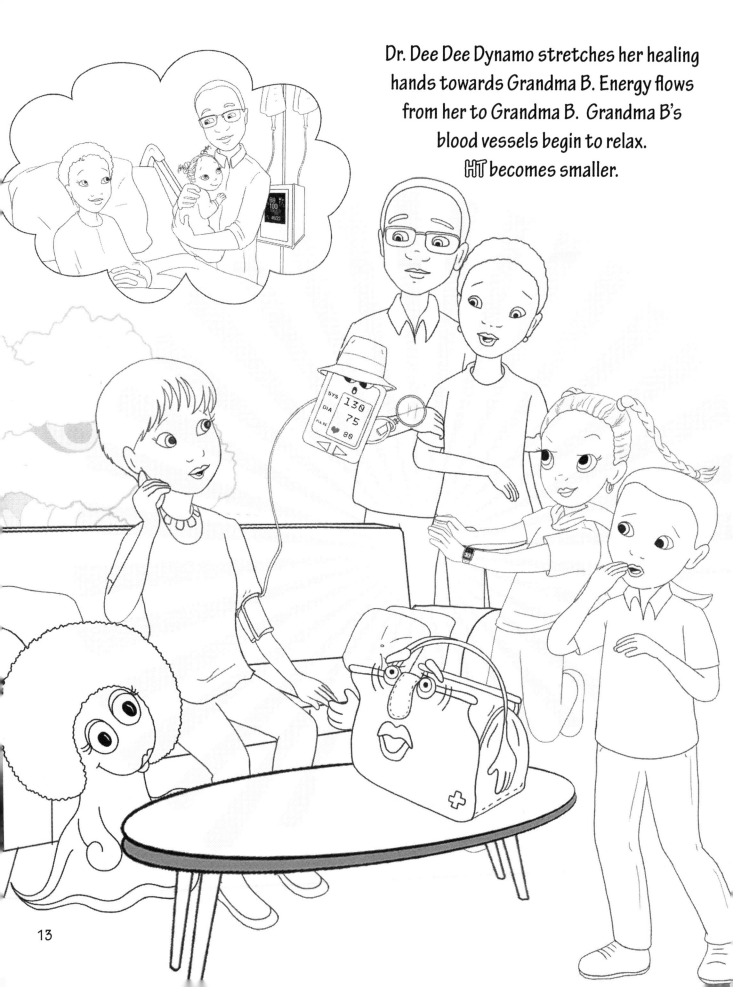

Dr. Dee Dee Dynamo stretches her healing hands towards Grandma B. Energy flows from her to Grandma B. Grandma B's blood vessels begin to relax. HT becomes smaller.

13

"Grandma B, did you take your medication this morning?"
Dr. Dee Dee asks gently.

"I got so busy and I felt fine," Grandma B says softly.
" I don't like taking the medicine because it sometimes makes me dizzy."

Mommy Dynamo says, " We will make an appointment to see your doctor."

"Why did HT attack Grandma B?" asks Lukas. "Is it because she's old?"

Mommy Dynamo explains. "HT can attack young and old.
Some of our food makes it easier for HT to get bigger."

"Grandma B's macaroni and cheese is filled with
Madame Soooo Dium's salty crystals. She helps HT grow!"

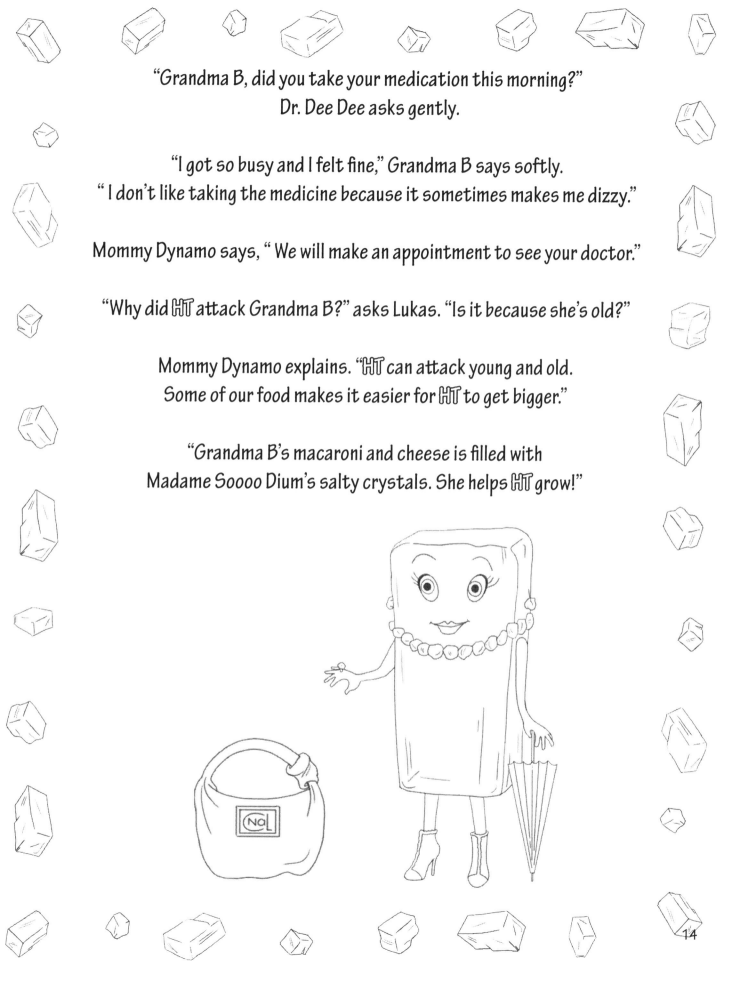

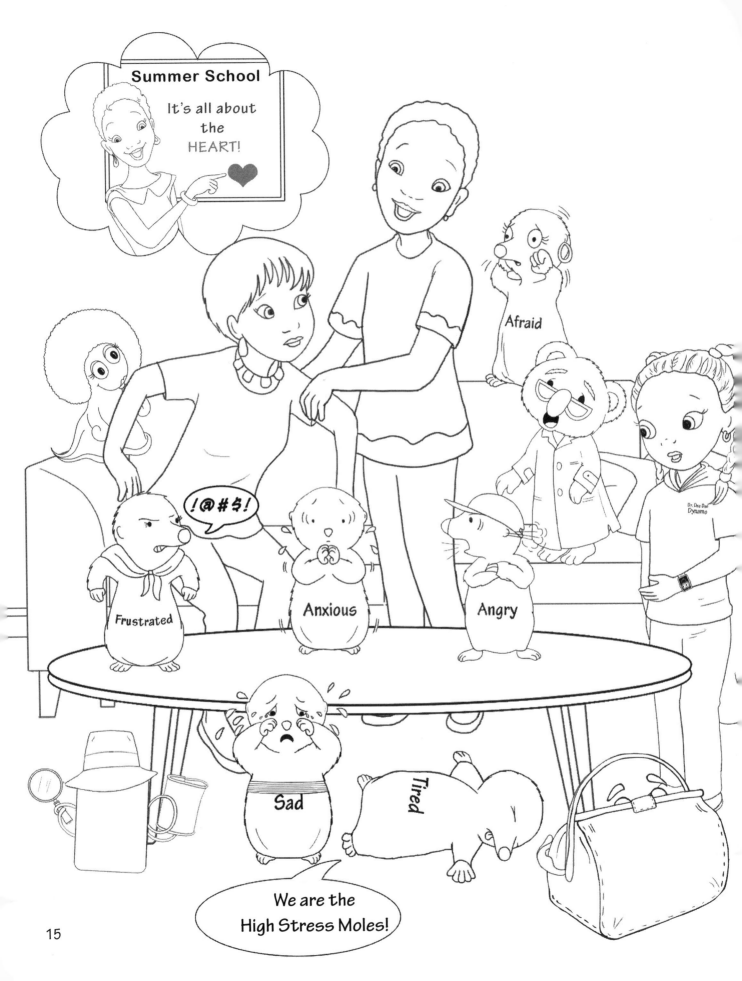

15

Norma Tension
aka
normal blood pressure

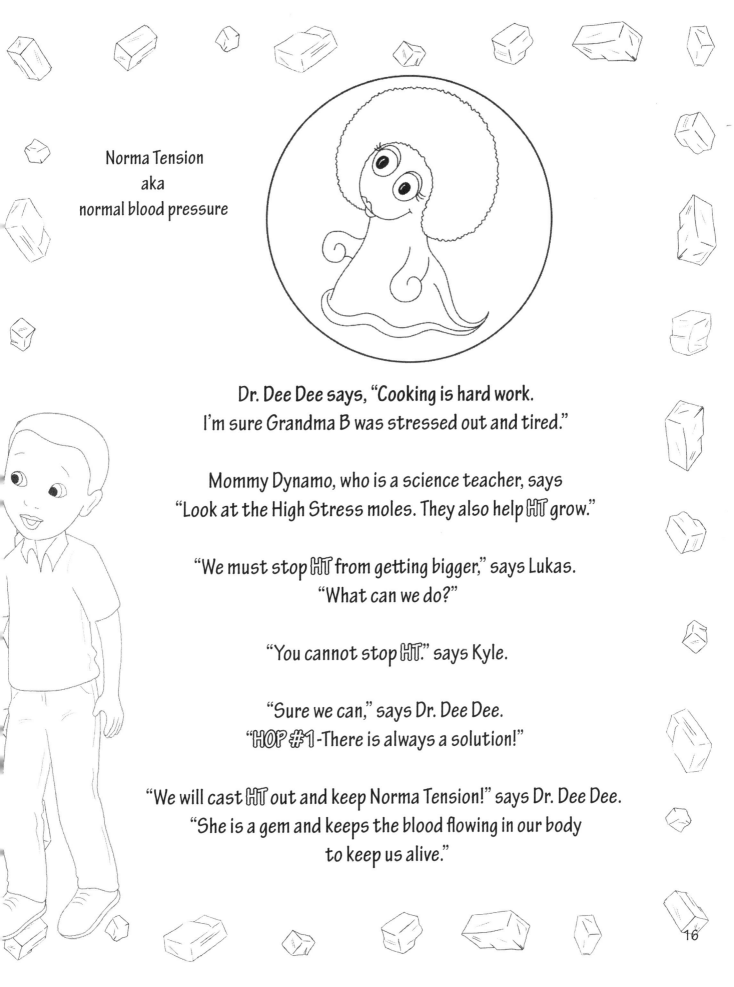

Dr. Dee Dee says, "Cooking is hard work.
I'm sure Grandma B was stressed out and tired."

Mommy Dynamo, who is a science teacher, says
"Look at the High Stress moles. They also help HT grow."

"We must stop HT from getting bigger," says Lukas.
"What can we do?"

"You cannot stop HT." says Kyle.

"Sure we can," says Dr. Dee Dee.
"HOP #1 -There is always a solution!"

"We will cast HT out and keep Norma Tension!" says Dr. Dee Dee.
"She is a gem and keeps the blood flowing in our body
to keep us alive."

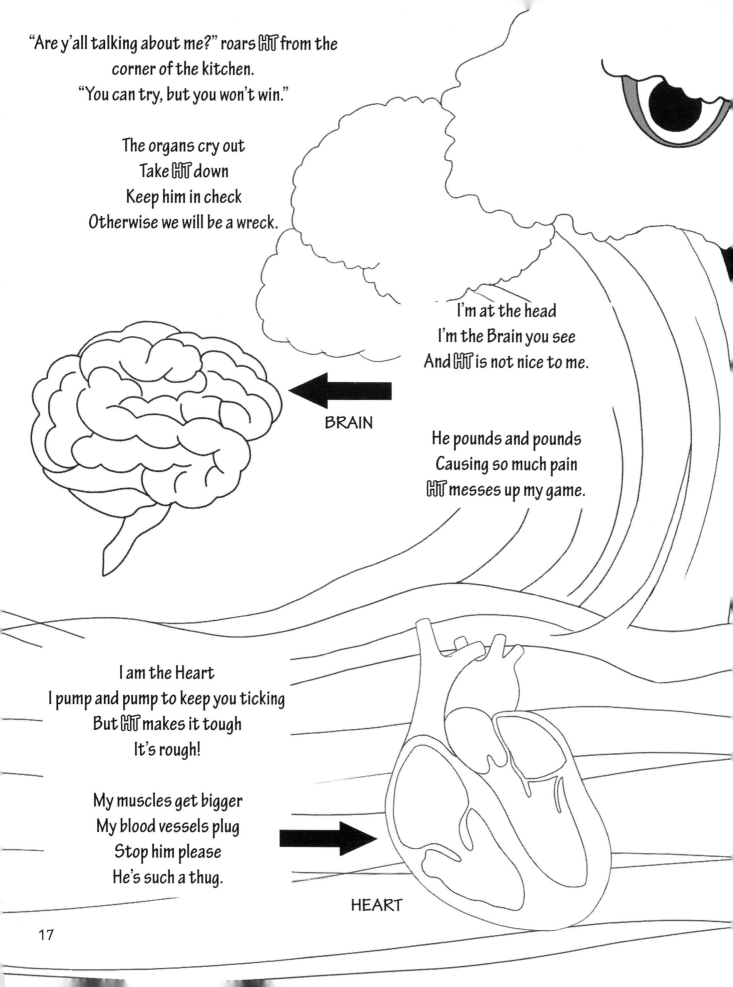

"Are y'all talking about me?" roars HT from the
corner of the kitchen.
"You can try, but you won't win."

The organs cry out
Take HT down
Keep him in check
Otherwise we will be a wreck.

I'm at the head
I'm the Brain you see
And HT is not nice to me.

BRAIN

He pounds and pounds
Causing so much pain
HT messes up my game.

I am the Heart
I pump and pump to keep you ticking
But HT makes it tough
It's rough!

My muscles get bigger
My blood vessels plug
Stop him please
He's such a thug.

HEART

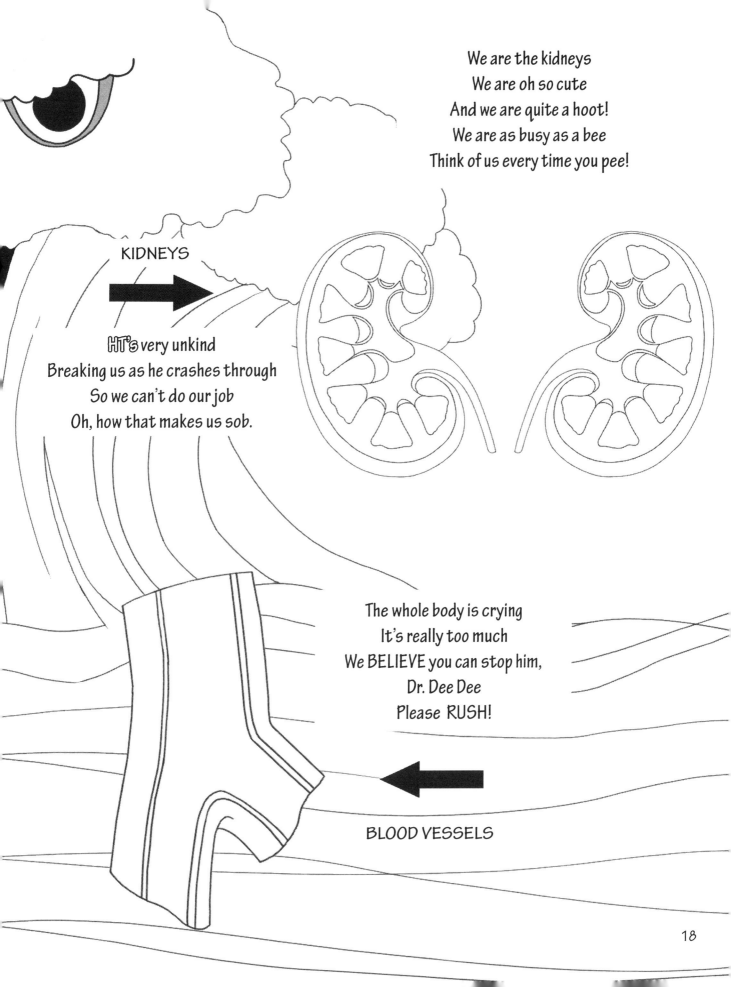

We are the kidneys
We are oh so cute
And we are quite a hoot!
We are as busy as a bee
Think of us every time you pee!

KIDNEYS

HT's very unkind
Breaking us as he crashes through
So we can't do our job
Oh, how that makes us sob.

The whole body is crying
It's really too much
We BELIEVE you can stop him,
Dr. Dee Dee
Please RUSH!

BLOOD VESSELS

18

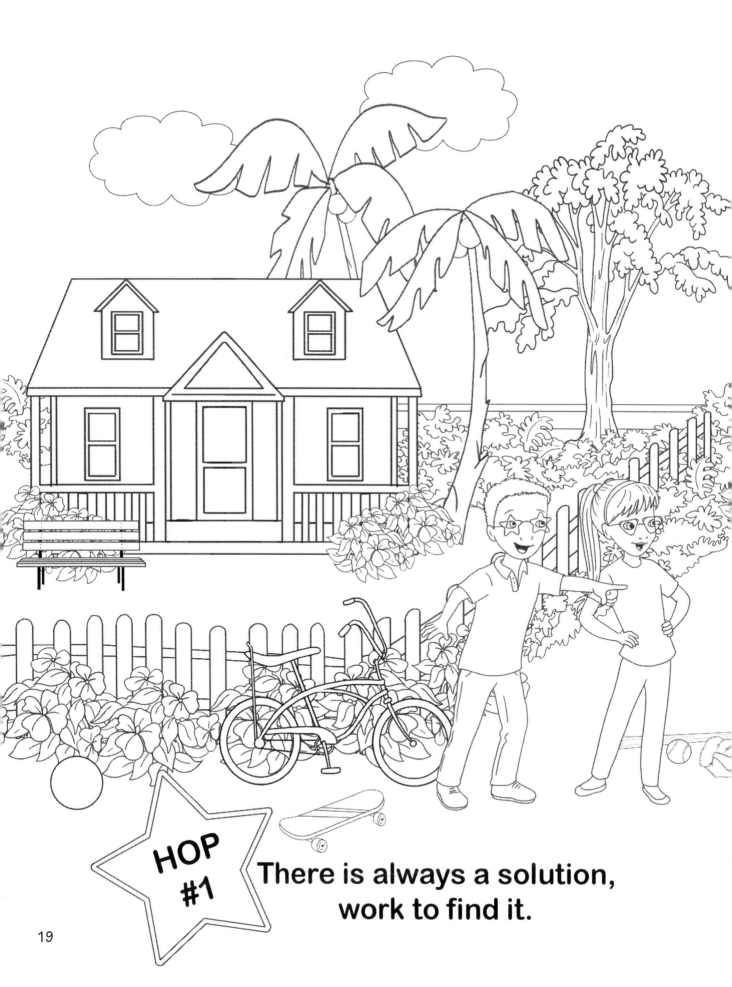

HOP #1

There is always a solution,
work to find it.

Let's go team, says Dr. Dee Dee
We have everything we need
There are no limits
We are going to succeed!

HOP to it with
Habit of Positivity #1
There is always a solution
We will work to find it
Taking down HT is going to be fun.

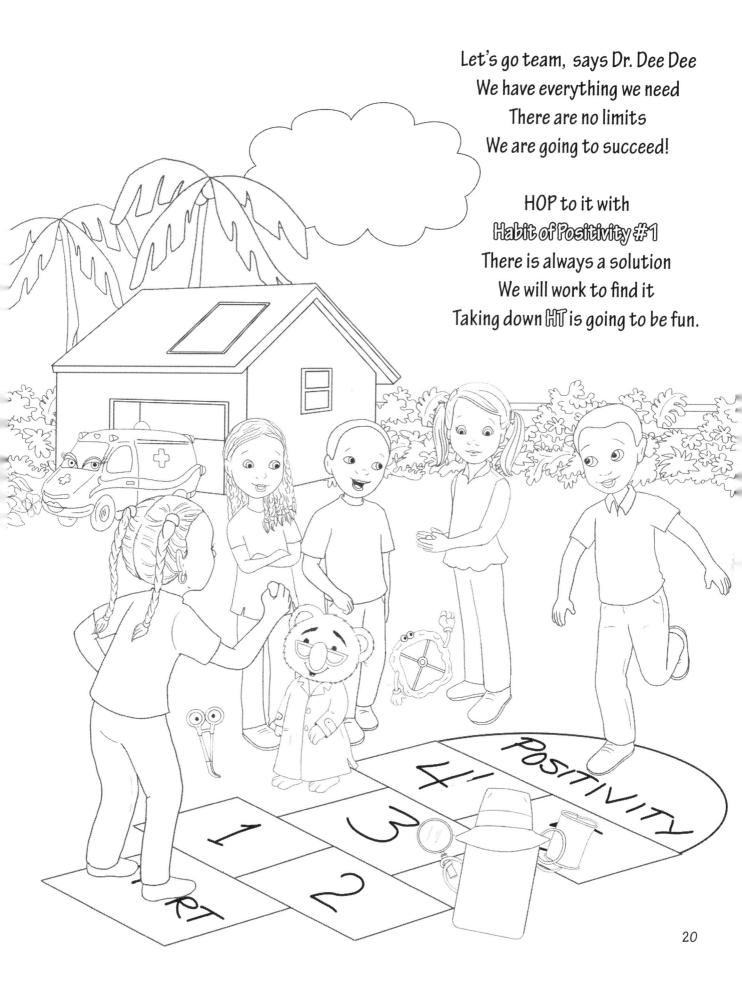

Not Even The Sky Is The Limit!

Dr. Dee Dee chants,
HT is a monster
A great big bully
But we've got his number
We will take him down, you'll see.

Bullies never win
Even if they seem big and strong
You have everything you need inside you
To win the battle all day long.

First we must find HT
Before he gets too large
He can run but he can't hide
We are in charge!

NEVER give up!

YOU ARE STRONG!

BE Courageous!

Bullies are cowards.

We can defeat them!

WORK TOGETHER!

HAVE FAITH!

Don't be afraid!

BELIEVE!

StayPositive!

Dr. Dee Dee Dynamo

Dr. Dee Dee says, "Bart Blood Pressure Cuff can help us find HT so we need to make lots of Barts."

"Freeda, set up the assembly line."

Kyle wrinkles his brow and complains. "How long is this going to take? I am exhausted."

Dr. Dee Dee encourages Kyle, "Hang in there buddy! You've got this!"

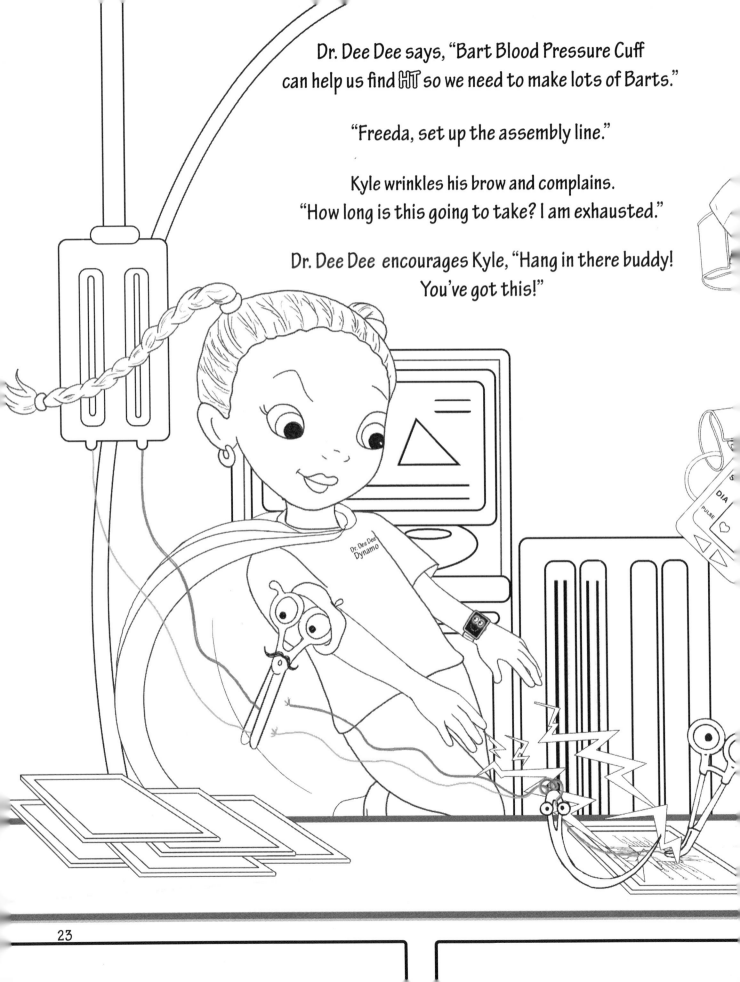

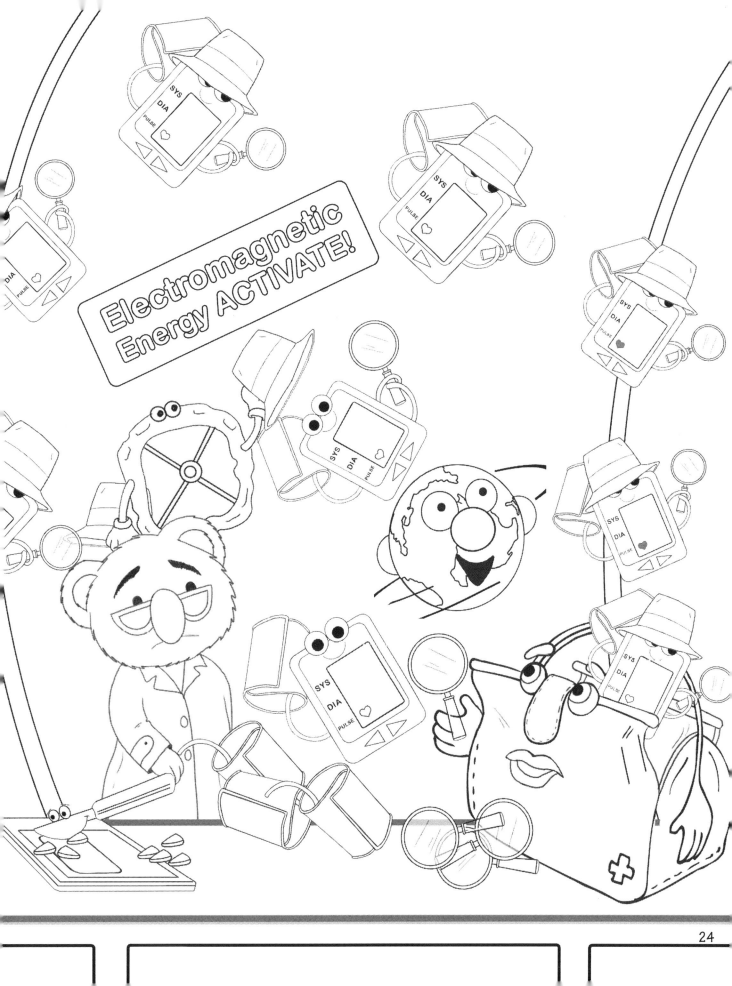

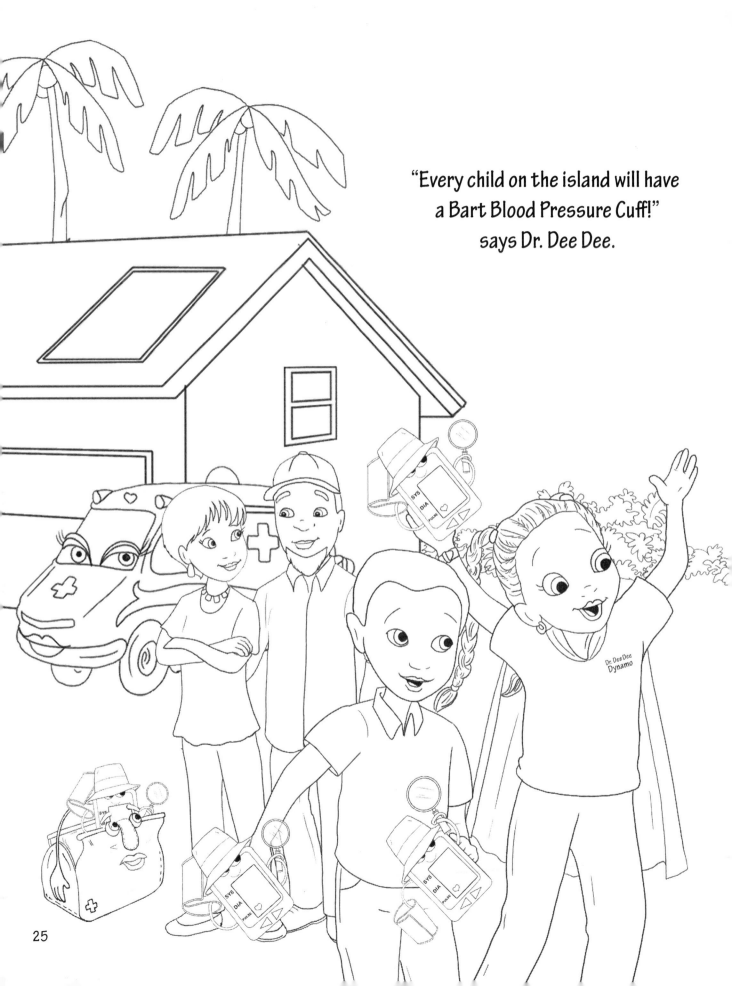

"Every child on the island will have a Bart Blood Pressure Cuff!" says Dr. Dee Dee.

25

"They will check blood pressures, beginning at home."

The young people pump Bart in the air and chant with excitement.
"BBPC Street Team reporting for duty!"

Lukas says. "We are coming for you HT!. Watch out!"

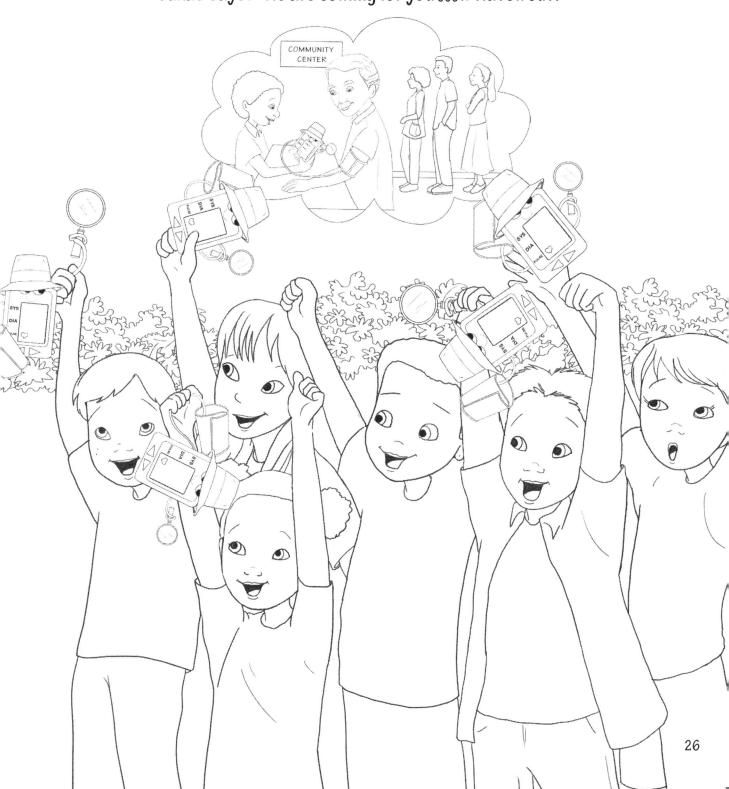

"We are not done Lukas," Dr. Dee Dee says. "Bart's Street Team cannot do it alone. We have other helpers who can help control HT."

"Meet the anti-HT crew:- Slum Ber, Take-Ur-Meds, Stress Buster, Low Salt, Exer & Cise, Good Nutrition and Mindful Mindy!!!"

"They work very well together so let's get them out there!"

Grandma B says, "They have really helped me. Thank you, Dr. Dee Dee."

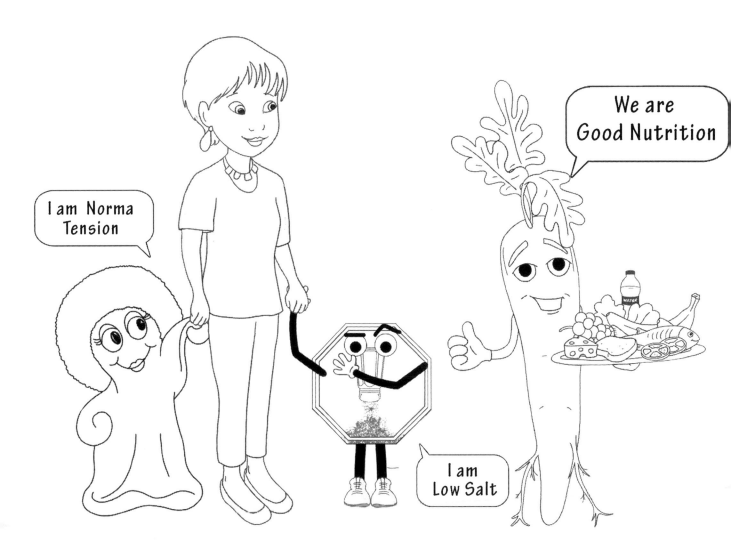

Anti-Hyper Tension Crew

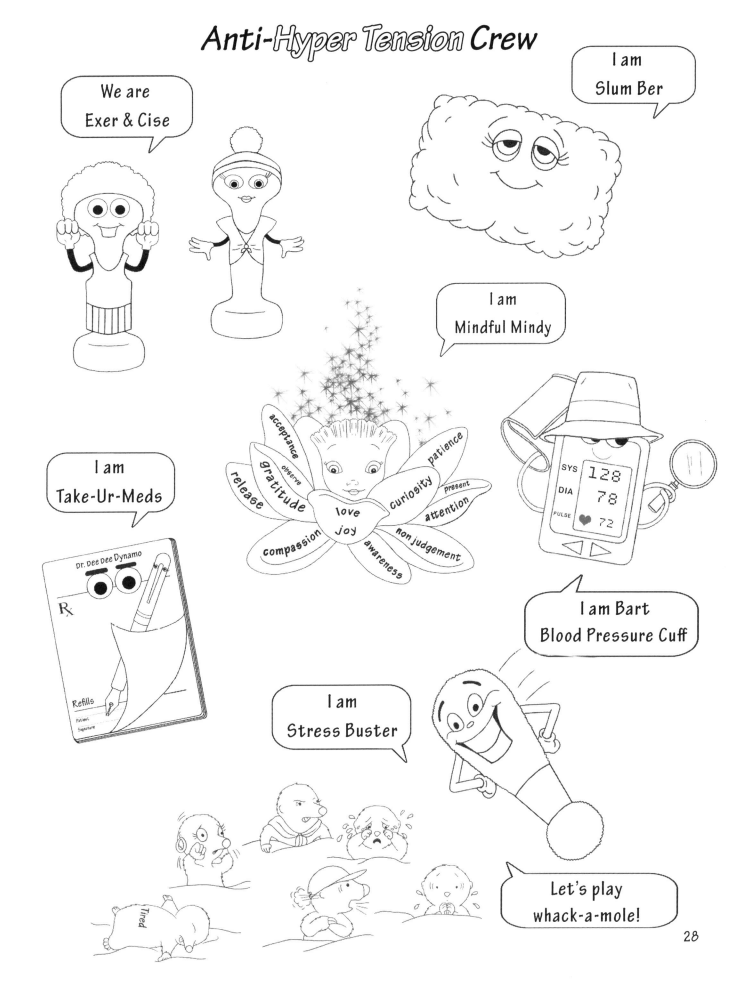

What We Do!

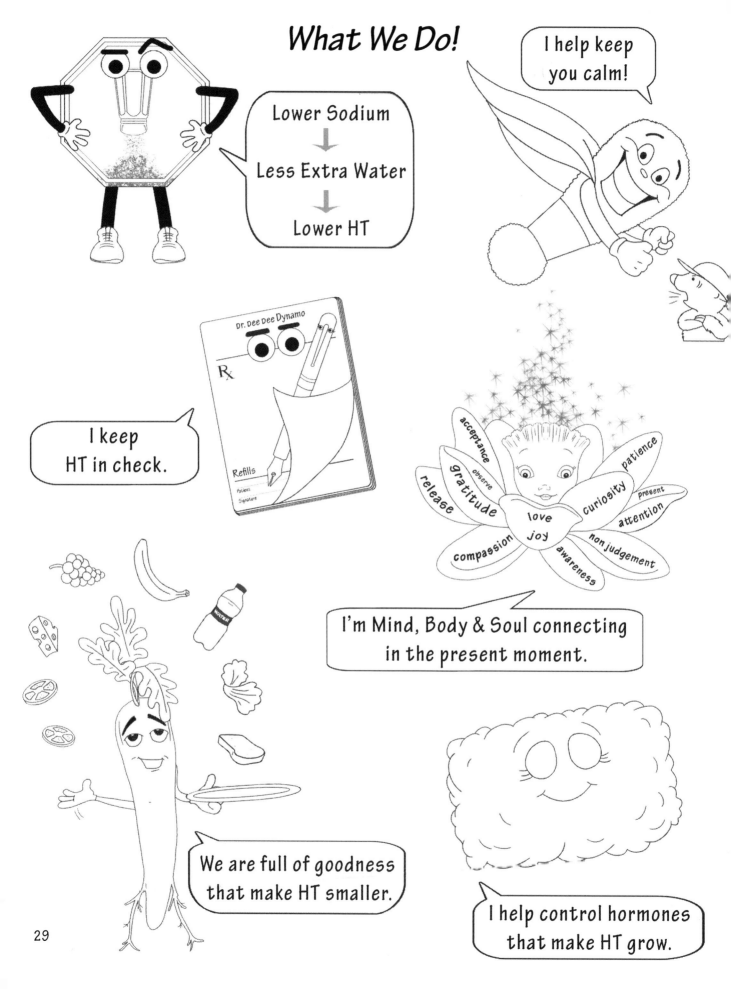

Dr. Dee Dee says, "Anti-HT Crew, you guys are great!"

"We love working with you, Dr. Dee Dee." Good Nutrition says.
"We are ready to take down that awful monster ⊞!!"

"Dr. Dee Dee, this is very exciting!" says Lukas . "We worked together and Grandma B
is doing better. Now, may we go back to the beach party?" he asks.

Kyle grumbles. "I say we cancel the party."

"No way, Kyle, the party must go on!" the team says, all at the same time.

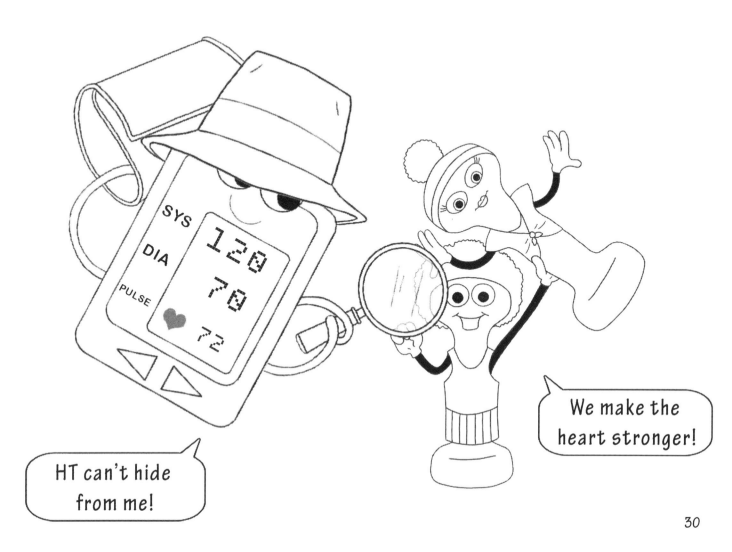

Dr. Dee Dee chuckles, "The party will go on! Good Nutrition has filled Freeda with loads of healthy foods and water. We will use Madame Soooo Dium in small amounts!" As Grandma B gets into Freeda, ℍ𝕋 tries to roar, but just a squeak comes out!

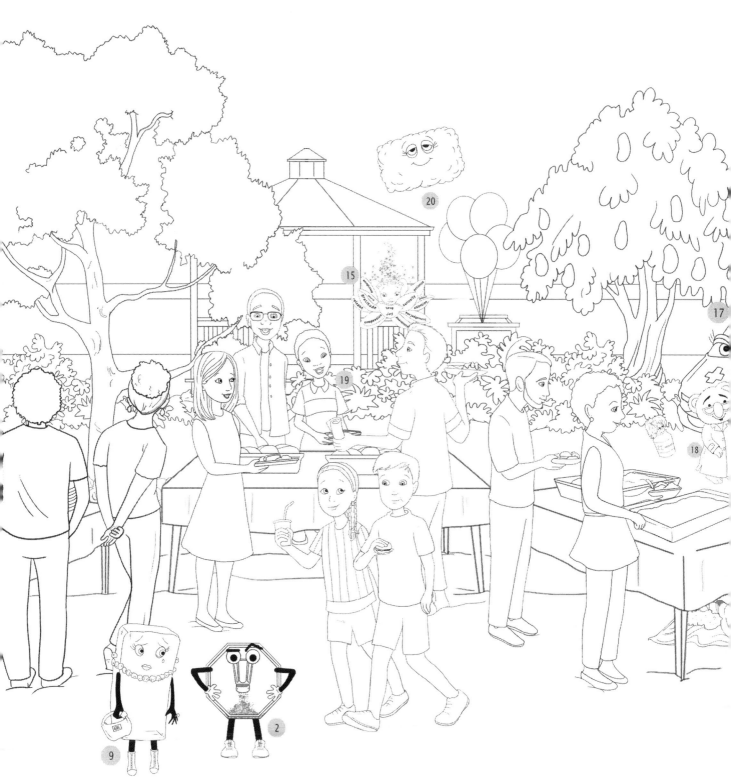

"Holymackarolee, Dr. Dee Dee!" exclaims Lukas, "I think we have taken HT down!"

Dr. Dee Dee is so happy! "Congratulations Team! You have been great! Because of you so many lives will be saved!" She says. "Let's stay on HT! Always remember to launch your Positivity Power through HOP #1 !!! There is always a solution and we worked together to find it!!!"

"Feel Good Beach!!! it's time to PARTY!!!!"

THE END

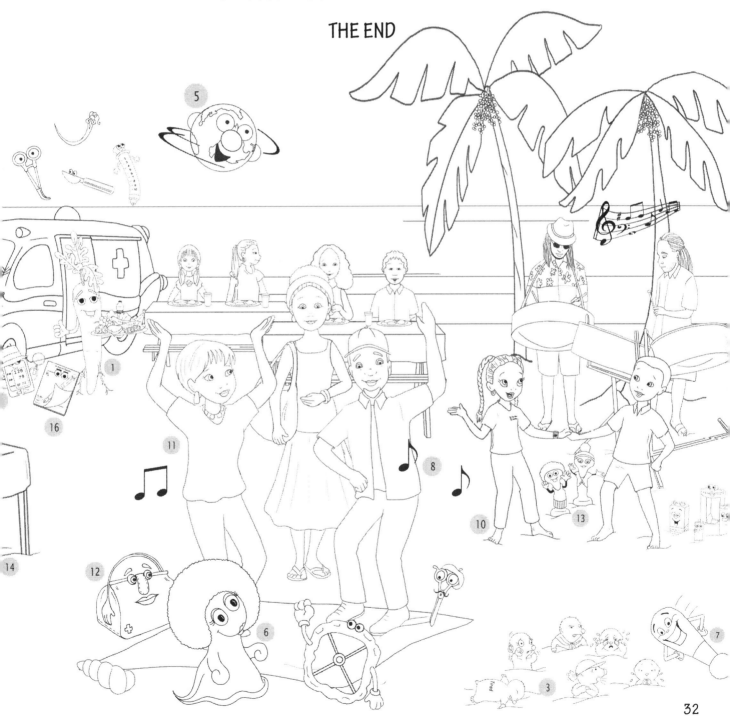

Tic- Tac- Toe

Character Scavenger Hunt

Match the numbers on page 31 and 32
to the characters listed below

1.____ Good Nutrition

2.____ Low Salt

3.____ High Stress Moles

4.____ Bart Blood Pressure Cuff

5.____ Gordon the Gullible Globe

6.____ Norma Tension

7.____ Stress Buster

8.____ Granddad Willy

9.____ Madame Soooo Dium

10.____ Dr. Dee Dee Dynamo

11.____ Grandma B

12.____ Marky Medicine Bag

13.____ Exer & Cise

14.____ Hyper Tension

15.____ Mindful Mindy

16.____ Take-Ur-Meds

17.____ Freeda the Flying Ambulance

18.____ Kyle the Koala Bear

19.____ Mommy Dynamo

20.____ Slum Ber

Answer Key

1. Dr Dee Dee Dynamo	6. Stress Buster	11. Bart Blood Pressure Cuff	16. Low Salt
2. Grandma B	7. Gordon the Gullible Globe	12. Exer & Cise	17. Mommy Dynamo
3. Granddad Willy	8. Madame Soooo Dium	13. Marky Medicine Bag	18. Kyle the Koala Bear
4. Norma Tension	9. Good Nutrition	14. Hyper Tension	19. Freeda the Flying Ambulance
5. High Stress Moles	10. Take-Ur-Meds	15. Slum Ber	20. Mindful Mindy

Hyper Tension Takedown Word Search

Words can be found in any direction (including diagonals) and can overlap each other. Use the word bank below.

```
T R A B F X W D E C N E I C S
O P U C F J S T R E S S C T S
H E U R B R A I N Q G X S D N
Z V V E X E R C I S E O B K B
F I A K M E U M D T R A E H M
R T L J S E V A M I N D F U L
E I G S G O D R S Y E N D I K
E S T X H Z S I E D O O L B M
D O M L H G E L C S I Y A V E
A P U E A J I Y E A E A Y D D
B T C B P S R H E S T R N R I
P E E L S G K Z J S S I P E T
S S N U T R I T I O N E O D A
G D V Z L C D Y N A M O V N T
M D N A L S I H A J E Q E P E
```

Word Bank

1. brain
2. high
3. dynamo
4. positive
5. heart
6. vessels
7. stress
8. exercise
9. medication
10. bart
11. kidneys
12. freeda
13. sleep
14. science
15. island
16. salt
17. eyes
18. mindful
19. nutrition
20. blood
21. meditate
22. preserve

What's my name?

Below is a list with the names of Dr. Dee Dee's team.
They help her to solve problems in the Universe.

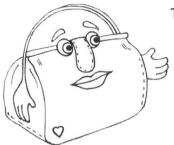

A) Freeda the Flying Ambulance
B) Gordon the Gullible Globe.
C) Kyle the Koala Bear
D) Marky Medicine Bag
E) Wyndee Watch

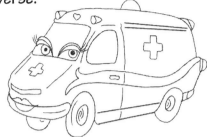

CLUES

1. Measures Dr. Dee Dee's electrical charge.

2. Carries Dr. Dee Dee's instruments.

3. Takes Dr. Dee Dee wherever she needs to go.

4. Is Dr. Dee Dee's grumpy assistant.

5. Has super sensitive ears, and sounds the alarm when someone is in distress.

NAMES

_____

_____

_____

_____

_____

Members of the Anti – HT crew are:

1. Exer & Cise
2. Slum Ber
3. Mindful Mindy
4. Take – Ur – Meds
5. Stress Buster
6. Bart Blood Pressure Cuff
7. Low Salt
8. Good Nutrition

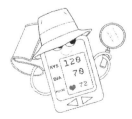

Answer the following:

Who...

A) Helps keep you calm ? _____

B) Measures blood pressure ? _____

C) Keeps HT in check ? _____

D) Controls hormones that make HT grow? _____

E) Connects you to the present moment ? _____

F) Helps the heart become stronger ? _____

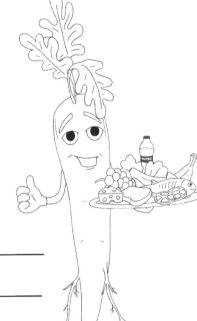

True or False

Select **True** or **False** for each statement below:

1) Madame Soooo Dium helps HT become stronger   T   F

2) A reading of 180/110 on Bart Blood Pressure Cuff is good   T   F

3) Stress makes HT lower   T   F

4) Good Nutrition can help control HT   T   F

5) The organs in the body love HT   T   F

Answers
1)T 2)F 3)F 4)T 5)F

All About Dr. Dee Dee Dynamo

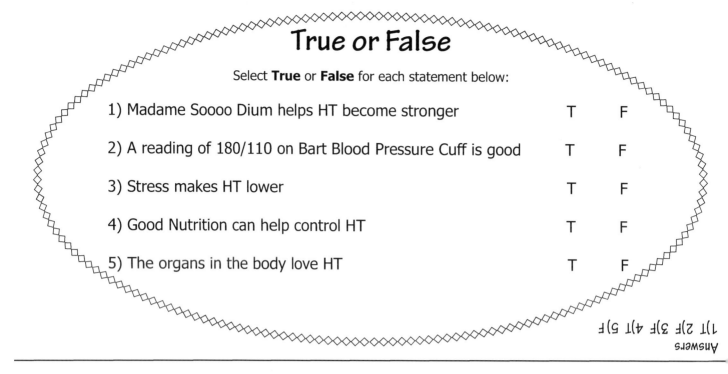

Across

3. Dr. Dee Dee and friends are dancing the _____

4. Dr. Dee Dee's hands are _____

5. Dr. Dee Dee doesn't have wings but she can _____

7. Dr. Dee Dee is ____ years old

10. Dr. Dee Dee is from the _____ of _____

13. Dr. Dee Dee's energy comes from _____ energy

14. Dr. Dee Dee loves to solve _____

Down

1. Dr. Dee Dee's Grandmother _____

2. Dr. Dee Dee's super power _____

6. Dr. Dee Dee's cousin _____

8. Dr. Dee Dee's mom is a _____

9. Dr. Dee Dee lives in _____

11. Dr. Dee Dee goes on missions with her _____

12. The color of Dr. Dee Dee's scrubs is _____

Answer Key:
Across: 3. Conga Line, 4. gifted, 5. fly, 7. nine, 10. Island of Positivity, 13. electrical, 14. problems
Down: 1. Grandma B., 2. positivity, 6. Lukas, 8. teacher, 9. Battery Grove, 11. team, 12. orange

Help Bart find HT

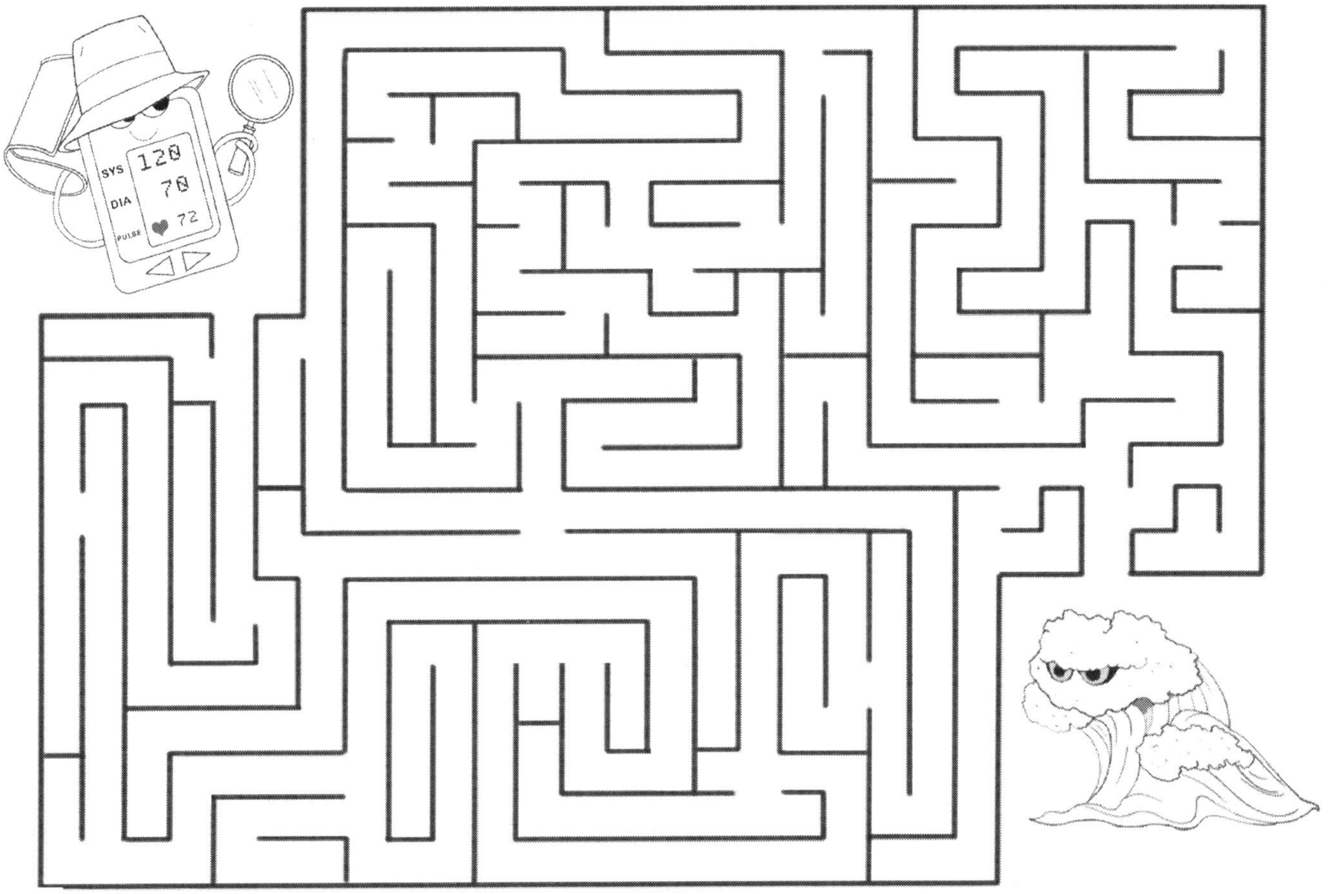

Unscramble these healthy food words and draw a line to their picture

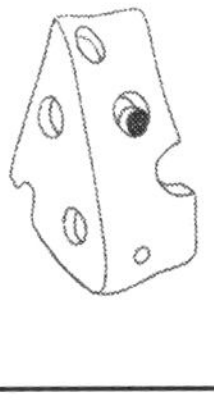

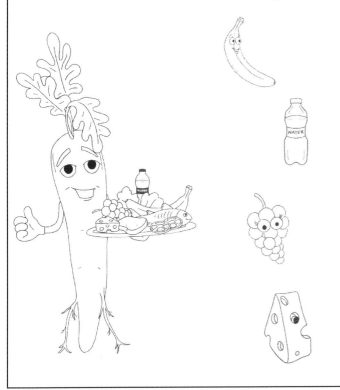

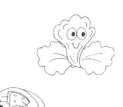

terwa ____________

uclette ____________

adebr ____________

sehece ____________

sprgae ____________

sihf ____________

naaban ____________

omatto ____________

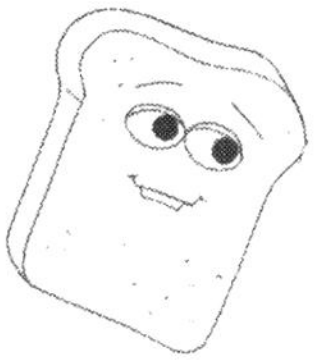

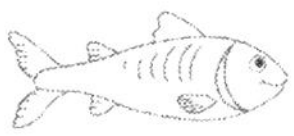

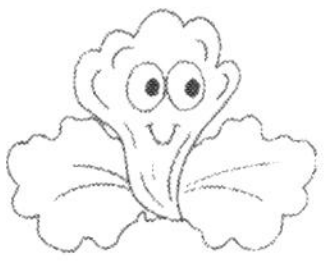

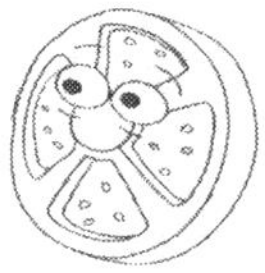

Answers: water, lettuce, bread, cheese, grapes, fish, banana, tomato

Connect the Dots

Name the characters

Trace and Color

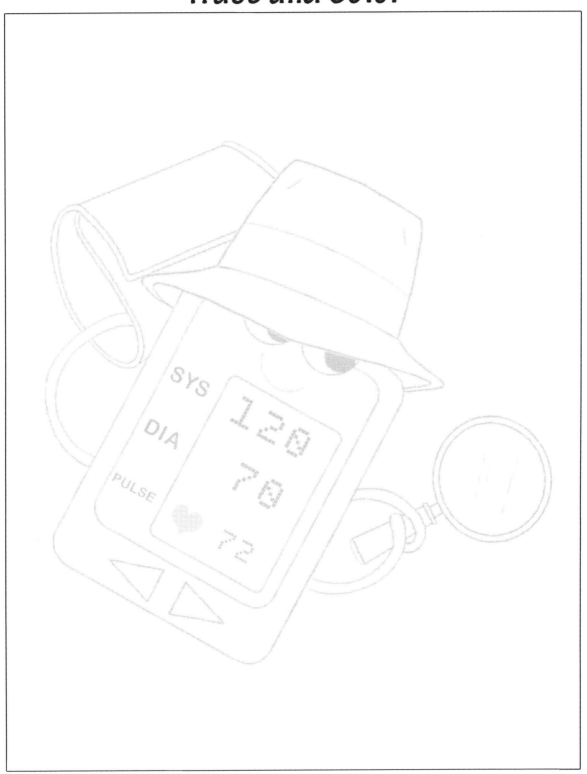

Trace and Color

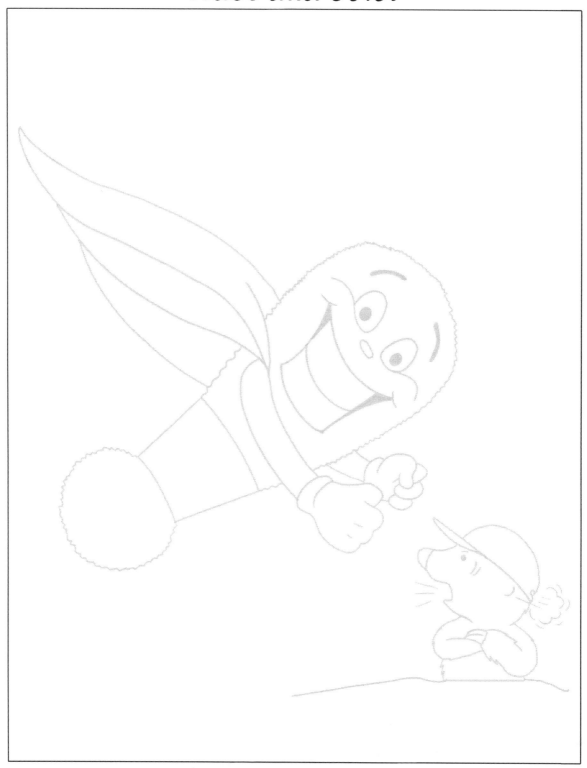

Trace and Color

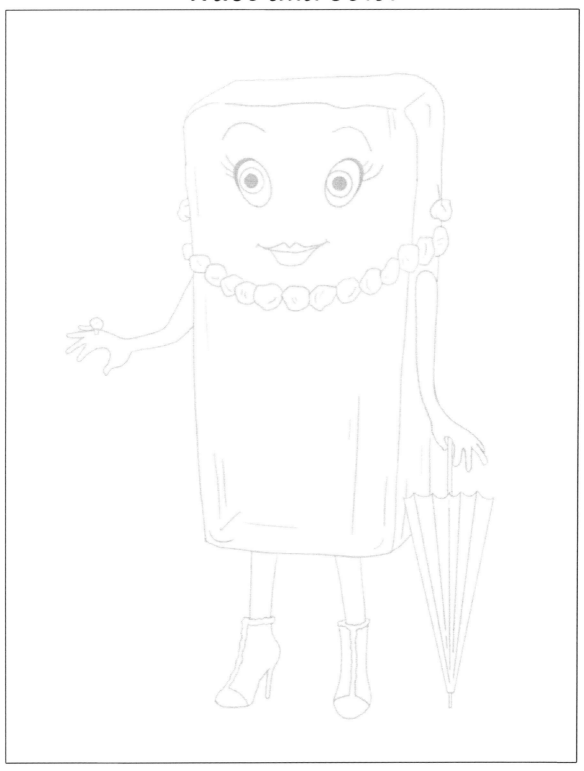

Trace and Color

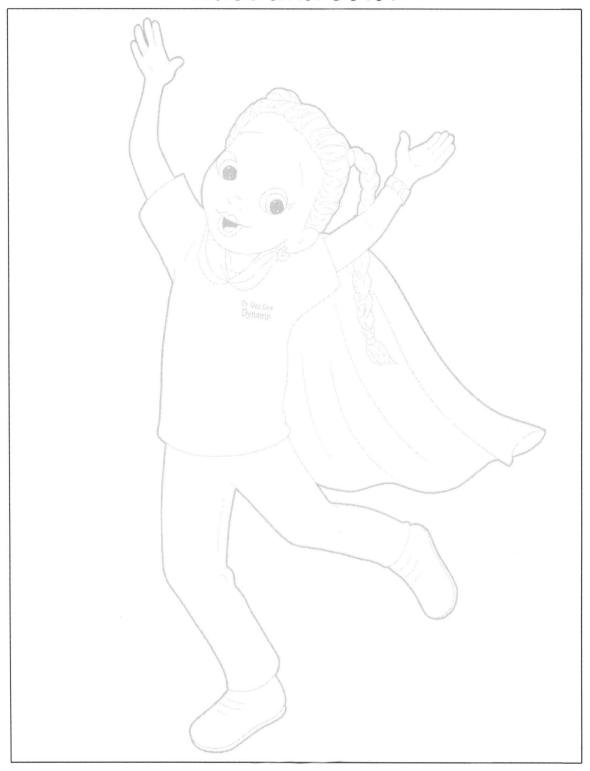

Trace and Color

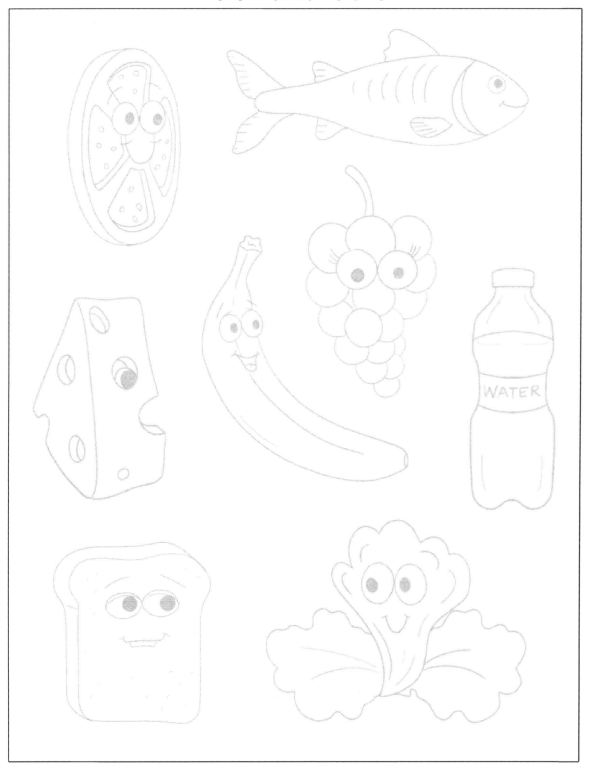

Welcome to the Positive Health Series!

My goal for this series is to highlight that we do have control over our health once we are 1)informed 2)understand the underlying issues involved and 3)BELIEVE that we can make choices that will positively impact our health. In addition, having a positive attitude makes a significant difference to our health by decreasing stress and helping us to be more proactive in how we take care of ourselves.

Hypertension, also known as high blood pressure, is a condition where the pressure in the blood vessels is elevated. As a result the heart works harder to pump the blood around the body. The increased pressure causes damage to the blood vessels in organs like the brain, eyes, heart and kidneys.

Hypertension is a major cause of death around the world with over 1 billion people affected. Yet, only half of those people are aware that their blood pressure is high. Less than 50% of those who know they have high blood pressure, are treated. In less wealthy countries, the percentage of people treated for high blood pressure is even lower and so there are more people who experience heart attacks, kidney disease and brain strokes.

IMAGINE if persons with hypertension were aware of its presence and received treatment. They would live longer and healthier lives!

IMAGINE if children used blood pressure cuffs regularly to check family members blood pressures. Hypertension could be identified before it became problematic and that would save lives!

IMAGINE if families read this book together. They would understand more about hypertension and be introduced to steps that can help prevent and manage hypertension. That would save lives!

IMAGINE if increased awareness and understanding as a result of reading this book caused people to visit their doctors or other health care providers, take their medications, make wise food choices, decrease salt, exercise, decrease stress and practice mindfulness! That would save lives!

IMAGINE approaching the problem with Habit of Positivity #1-There is always a solution, we CAN find it! First we must acknowledge the problem, turn it upside down to understand it and then work together to create solutions that will SAVE LIVES!

Don't let the Hyper Tension monster win! We CAN take him down!

Dr. Oneeka Williams

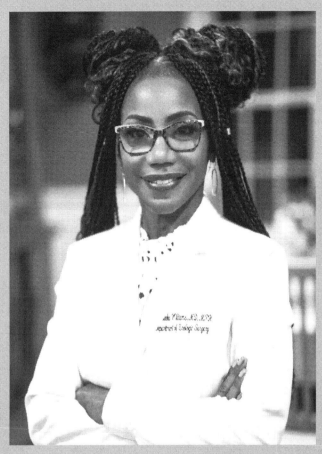

DR. ONEEKA WILLIAMS IS A STORYTELLER, SURGEON AND POSITIVITY CATALYST WHO GREW UP IN THE CARIBBEAN. HER MOTHER, A SCIENCE TEACHER, AND FATHER, A JOURNALIST BOTH CONTRIBUTED TO HER EARLY LOVE OF SCIENCE AND WRITING.

AT AGE 13, DR. WILLIAMS DECIDED THAT SHE WAS GOING TO BE A DOCTOR. WHEN SHE FIRST ENTERED THE OPERATING ROOM WHILE ATTENDING HARVARD MEDICAL SCHOOL, IT WAS LOVE AT FIRST SIGHT AND SHE WORKED HARD TO ACHIEVE HER DREAM OF BECOMING A SURGEON.

IF SHE COULD DO IT,

DR. DEE DEE DYNAMO IS DR. WILLIAMS' VEHICLE TO EDUCATE, ELEVATE AND EMPOWER THE NEXT GENERATION TO DREAM BIG, BE HEALTHY, LOVE SCIENCE AND READING, AND LIVE A LIFE WITHOUT LIMITS!

SHE IS A PRACTICING SURGEON OUTSIDE BOSTON WHERE SHE LIVES WITH HER HUSBAND, CHARLES AND SON, MARK.

THIS IS THE FIRST BOOK IN THE DR. DEE DEE DYNAMO POSITIVE HEALTH SERIES.

YOU CAN FIND THE OTHER TITLES IN THE DR. DEE DEE DYNAMO BOOK SERIES AT WWW.DRDEEDEEDYNAMO.COM

Family Blood Pressure Chart

Date Name	Sun. BP	Mon. BP	Tues. BP	Wed. BP	Thurs. BP	Fri. BP	Sat. BP

Blood Pressure Levels

Normal - less than 120/80 mm Hg
Prehypertension -120-139/80-89
Hypertension - greater than 140/90 mm Hg

Made in the USA
Columbia, SC
26 November 2024

46591733R00030